YOUR KNOWLEDGE HAS VALUE

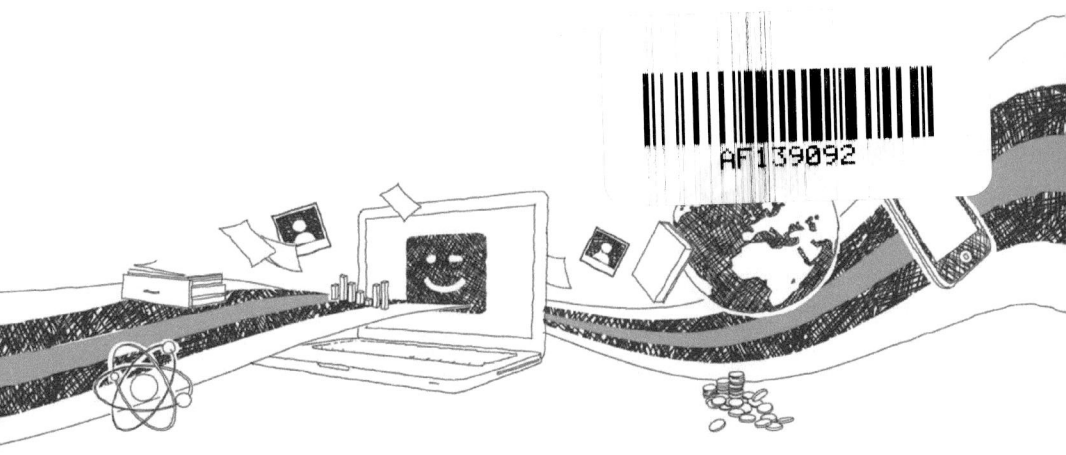

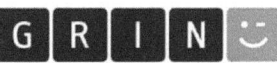

Bibliographic information published by the German National Library:

The German National Library lists this publication in the National Bibliography; detailed bibliographic data are available on the Internet at http://dnb.dnb.de .

Imprint:

Copyright © 2007 GRIN Verlag
Print and binding: Books on Demand GmbH, Norderstedt Germany
ISBN: 9783668960398

This book at GRIN:

https://www.grin.com/document/475182

Timothy John Whittard

Interprofessional collaboration in the healthcare industry. The benefits of getting it right and the dangers of getting it wrong.

GRIN Verlag

GRIN - Your knowledge has value

Since its foundation in 1998, GRIN has specialized in publishing academic texts by students, college teachers and other academics as e-book and printed book. The website www.grin.com is an ideal platform for presenting term papers, final papers, scientific essays, dissertations and specialist books.

Visit us on the internet:

http://www.grin.com/

http://www.facebook.com/grincom

http://www.twitter.com/grin_com

Trigger

"When registered I will be working to achieve interprofessional partnerships. How will I manage accountability to different bosses and to the consumer/user/patient?" (Anon, 2006).

The following briefing paper aims to discuss and explore the issues raised by the above trigger and my subsequent reading around the issue of 'accountability'; personal thoughts and feelings will be cited in order to clarify and individualise the opinions and arguments provoked. First it may be beneficial to examine the meaning of the term 'accountability'. It is reported by Kupperschmidt (2004) that this pertains to "being responsible" to oneself and others for "behaviours and outcomes" included in the "professional role" of an individual; Brinkerhoff (2003) elaborates, highlighting that accountability also carries an "obligation of individuals or agencies to provide information about" and also "justification" for their actions.

Professionals are accountable "in many areas" or their work (Bothamley, 2006) and all staff members are personally accountable for their own practice, including any "casual mistakes or deliberate abuse" (Martin, 2001). Importantly, it is acknowledged by Brinkerhoff (2003) that with accountability there coexists an inherent risk for potential consequences for individual professionals in terms of "answerability" and "legal procedures"; adding that such risks to the individual practitioner are "at the core of enforcing accountability".

Obviously the need for accountability is unquestionable within the healthcare system, where mistakes can have the potential to cause "wrongful death or injury" to patients (Reid, 2004); however, as a student nurse I find the anticipation and prospect of handling such responsibility post-registration can be massively daunting and the source of much anxiety. According to Bothamley (2006) I am not alone; she suggests

1

that many student healthcare professionals do not feel or appear to be fully prepared "for professional practice and the responsibility that this involves". This highlights personal doubts regarding my own professional abilities and also a lack of confidence. In addition, it is interesting to note that Reid (2004) states that some professional titles "may infer duties and standards" that the title-holder is unaware of or unable to fulfil; this emphasises a real need for professionals to understand exactly what they are "accountable for" and "to whom" (Martin, 2001). Consequently, Cohen (2004) reports that individual professionals must be clear about what is expected of them; adding that such a lack of clarity regarding accountability presents a "common obstacle" to successful interprofessional collaboration.

During clinical practice I will endeavour to seek complete comprehension of my accountabilities to ensure that I am able to successfully meet the expectations of my role; there are probably few, if any, healthcare professionals who have not at one time or another failed to rise to their accountabilities (Reid, 2004) and I feel that a personal recognition of the potential for being held accountable for tragedy and lawsuits will serve to motivate my practice.

Despite this, Martin (2001) reports that whilst professionals must possess sufficient confidence to perform effectively, they must also acknowledge the limitations of their abilities and personal resources, in order to ensure that "they seek support when necessary". This approach to practice is currently inherent in my role as a student healthcare professional, where I am required to be supervised in my learning and practice; however, I feel that continuing to seek support and input from fellow professionals, across different disciplines will be beneficial to the management of my personal accountabilities.

Reference List

Brinkerhoff, D. (2003) *Accountability and Health Systems: Overview, Framework, and Strategies.* Bethesda, Maryland: Partners for Health Reform*plus.* – [online] Available from: http://www.phrplus.org/pubs/tech018_fin.pdf.

Bothamley, J. (2006) Face up to responsibility. *Nursing Standard* 20(45) p.77.

Cohen, S. (2004) The push and pull of staff accountability. *Nursing Management* 35(6) p.10.

Kupperschmidt, B. (2004) Making a Case for Shared Accountability. *Journal of Nursing Administration* 34(3) p.114-116.

Martin, V. (2001) Service planning and governance: Part Two: Managing accountability and risk. *Nursing Management* 8(3) p.33-37.

Reid, W. (2004) Organization Liability: Beyond *Respondeat Superior. Journal of Psychiatric Practice* 10(4) p.258-262.

This briefing paper is aimed at the members of my interprofessional module group, and intends to extend the discussion of the preceding briefing paper by further exploring issues surrounding the management of professional accountability within the healthcare system; opening the debate to include the subjects of clinical governance, patient-centred care, and collaborative practice. Personal experience will be used in order to highlight and reinforce significant aspects of the discussion.

As mentioned previously, the term 'accountability' refers to the complex responsibilities of individual professionals, to various parties, which are inherently attached to their professional identity (Brinkerhoff, 2003; and Kupperschmidt, 2004). It is reported by Bothamley (2006) that making the transition from a student to a qualified healthcare professional can be, for many, a daunting prospect due to the challenges presented by an increase in professional accountability; this view is reiterated by Nancarrow and Mackey (2005) who highlight that although the working practices of student healthcare professionals may be no different to those of their qualified counterparts, there are significant increases in accountability post-registration. As a student nurse my accountabilities after qualifying will be legally enforced by a professional code of conduct (NMC, 2004).

A recent influx of government policies and initiatives detail 'clinical governance' as a key milestone on the road to improved care delivery; this concept places responsibility on all individual professionals for the continued and sustained development and improvement of service provision (Checkland et al, 2004; DOH, 1998; and Wilkinson et al, 2004). Clinical governance serves as a measure to prevent mistakes, abuse and misconduct (Martin, 2001; and Onion, 2000).

Despite this, it is interesting to note that the demand on the health services to meet government guidelines can cause difficulties to arise whereby practitioners are torn between their accountability to their organisation and the achieving of targets, and their accountability to the patient (Cranwell and Buchanan, 2005; and Halligan and Donaldson, 2001); consequently, there may be occasions when accountability to patients is overlooked, as organisational accountability is prioritised (Onion, 2000). I

4

have witnessed an example of this during clinical practice, where a detained patient in a psychiatric intensive care unit was prescribed only escorted leave from the hospital grounds, meaning that they could not leave the ward or go outdoors unless accompanied by staff; the patient wished to go outside for some fresh air and a change of scenery, and had waited patiently for several hours, yet ward staff were not able to facilitate the request in a timely fashion. The ward staff were not only accountable to the inpatients on their ward, but were also accountable to the rest of the hospital for carrying medical emergency response equipment, and did not have the necessary staff numbers to both escort the patient and cover the hospital for the event of a medical emergency.

According to the DOH (2006) if healthcare professionals are to deliver effective and holistic care then a patient-centred approach must be adopted. Although, this notion is widely recognised and is reiterated throughout numerous recent government publications and professional journals, it is not always achieved with consistency in practice (Fulford et al, 1996). There are many factors, which can obstruct the successful implementation of a patient-centred approach; however, Hogston et al (2002) suggest that there is a need for the development of comprehensive policies which place the patient at the focus of clinical practice and raise accountability to patients to the top of the workplace agenda.

It is reported by both Headrick et al (1998) and Hornby and Atkins (2000) that with increasingly complex patient needs, the delivery of effective holistic care is rarely the province of only one professional group; this emphasises the unquestionable need for professionals to collaborate in the delivery of care to meet the growing diverse and involved needs of patients. One may assume that a need to collaborate across professional disciplines and agencies is also implicit of a need for professionals to actively develop and sustain interprofessional relationships with their colleagues and fellow team members in order to ensure the success of this process.

Significantly, Hewison and Sim (1998) state that professional codes of conduct for all healthcare disciplines dictate that interprofessional collaboration must form the backbone of practice, asserting that qualified practitioners possess a legal and ethical requirement to adopt an interprofessional approach to practice. However, as discussed this is not a clean-cut process, and in order to facilitate smooth and successful collaboration professionals must be clear about their accountabilities (Martin, 2001) and seek guidance with them when necessary (Reid, 2004; and

Wilkinson et al, 2004). I feel that writing this briefing paper has allowed me to acquire a useful knowledge and understanding of the intricacies of professional accountability and how it will effect my future practice as a qualified professional.

Word count – 791.

6

Reference List

Brinkerhoff, D. (2003) *Accountability and Health Systems: Overview, Framework, and Strategies.* Bethesda, Maryland: Partners for Health Reform*plus.* – [online] Available from: http://www.phrplus.org/pubs/tech018_fin.pdf.

Bothamley, J. (2006) Face up to responsibility. *Nursing Standard* 20(45) p.77.

Carnwell, R. and Buchanan, J. (2005) *Effective Practice in Health and Social Care: A Partnership Approach.* Maidenhead: Open University Press.

Checkland, K., Marshall, M. and Harrison, S. (2004) Re-thinking accountability: trust versus confidence in medical practice. *Quality & Safety in Health Care* 13 p.130-135.

DOH (1998) *A First Class Service, Quality in the NHS.* London: Stationary Office.

DOH (2006) *Essence of Care: Benchmarks for Promoting Health.* London: Department of Health.

Fulford, K., Ersser, S. and Hope, T. (1996) *Essential Practice in Patient-Centred Care.* London: Blackwell Science.

Halligan, A. and Donaldson, L. (2001) Implementing clinical governance: turning vision into reality. *British Medical Journal* 322 p.1413-1417.

Headrick, L., Wilcock, P. and Batalden, P. (1998) Continuing medical education: Interprofessional working and continuing medical education. *British Medical Journal* 316(7133) p.771-774.

Hewison, A. and Sim, J. (1998) Managing interprofessional working: using codes of ethics as a foundation. *Journal of Interprofessional Care* 12(3) p.309-321.

Hogston, R. and Simpson, P. (2002*) Foundations of Nursing Practice. Making the Difference.* 2nd ed. Hampshire: Palgrave Macmillan.

Hornby, S. and Atkins, J. (2000) *Collaborative Care: Interprofessional, Interagency and Interpersonal.* 2nd ed, Oxford: Blackwell Science.

Kupperschmidt, B. (2004) Making a Case for Shared Accountability. *Journal of Nursing Administration* 34(3) p.114-116.

Martin, V. (2001) Service planning and governance: Part Two: Managing accountability and risk. *Nursing Management* 8(3) p.33-37.

Nancarrow, S. and Mackey, H. (2005) The introduction and evaluation of an occupational therapy assistant practitioner. *Australian Occupational Therapy Journal* 52 p.293-301.

NMC (2004) The NMC code of professional conduct: standards for conduct, performance and ethics.

Onion, C. (2000) Principles to Govern Clinical Governance. *Journal of Evaluation in Clinical Practice* 6(4) p.405-412.

Reid, W. (2004) Organization Liability: Beyond *Respondeat Superior*. *Journal of Psychiatric Practice* 10(4) p.258-262.

Wilkinson, J., Rushmore, R. and Davies, H. (2004) Clinical governance and the learning organisation. *Journal of Nursing Management* 12 p.105-113 .

This following document is a report that aims to critique a briefing paper, which was produced by a fellow member of the interprofessional module. The critique criteria devised by my interprofessional group during an earlier task will be employed as a framework to guide the writing of this document.

The briefing paper that is being examined states its aims and focus directly, making clear its purpose within the opening paragraph; progressing to provide details of the chosen subject matter, and the areas covered in the pending discussion. According to Wilkie (2007) this is important, as a briefing paper should "inform the reader about its subject quickly and effectively"; therefore allowing the reader to ascertain how useful or relevant the paper is to their needs. The author also explains the origins of their briefing paper, and how it was developed from previous academic work. This furnishes the briefing paper with transparency regarding the intentions of its author, allowing the reader to observe and understand the goals of the writer.

The introductory elements of this paper state that 'clinical governance' is intended to be a key and focal concept for the discussion of the paper; however, although the context of the issues raised throughout the paper are in keeping with the central theme, it may have been possible to maintain this as the focus more often. Also, it may be worth noting that whilst the topic of 'clinical governance' is cited as an area of significance and the rationale for this is provided, little attention is given to defining this term or concept.

It is suggested by the author that the issues raised within the briefing paper may be of a greater concern to healthcare professionals at "junior level", perhaps implying that the intended audience of this paper is to be student healthcare professionals; however, beyond this it is not immediately clear who the paper is aimed at. This is significant, as Fiske (1990, p.74) reports that if an author wishes their work to "receive the mass reception it needs, it must deal with matters of general concern" to a specific audience. Importantly, despite this, the author does acknowledge the discussions of the preceding briefing papers and does not excessively or unnecessarily repeat their content, demonstrating an awareness of previous or existing knowledge that the reader may possess. Additionally, the structure of the paper flows easily and is written in an appropriate coherent, fluent and professional language style, which reflects the academic nature of the paper and allows the reader to follow the thoughts of the author without confusion (National AIDs Manual, 2002).

A wide range of supporting literature is used throughout the briefing paper in order to provide balanced and unbiased arguments, and to reinforce a series of interesting and thought-provoking viewpoints; the author does make some assumptions during the course of the paper, however these are largely supported by the literature. Despite this, there are occasions in the text where the writer does not support their claims as fully as perhaps possible, and additionally there is also little evidence to suggest that the author has critically appraised the source material. Importantly, according to the National AIDs Manual (2002) a sufficient quantity of references has been employed, and all sources used throughout the briefing paper are detailed in the reference list according to the 'Harvard' method of referencing. It may also be worth noting that although all supporting literature is referenced appropriately, the correct format for doing so is not utilised as rigorously as possible by the author, for example the reference list is not arranged into alphabetical order (BMA, 2007).

The briefing paper does explore the topic of 'clinical governance', which pertains to one of the specified module themes; the paper also achieves the criteria of the relevant learning outcomes, discussing the impact of one of the specified issues upon the quality of care, which is delivered. Within the briefing paper opposing views are well presented, and ideas and arguments are challenged, with recommendations from the author being provided. The author also acknowledges the implications of ethical issues, when discussing the duty of care to patients. The paper is both informative and interesting, and is summarised clearly and succinctly; additionally the aims as outlined in the "statement of purpose" (Wilkie, 2007) are largely fulfilled.

The process of critiquing this work has been beneficial, by allowing the opportunity to acquire an understanding of this subject from the viewpoint of a fellow student healthcare professional of a different discipline.

Word count – 747.

11

Reference List

BMA (2007) *Information factsheets - Reference styles.* London: British Medical Association. – [online] Available from:
http://www.bma.org.uk/ap.nsf/Content/LIBReferenceStyles
[Accessed 18th December 2007].

Fiske, J. (1990) *Introduction to Communication Studies.* London: Routledge.

National AIDs Manual (2002) *Advocacy card - Preparing a briefing note or position paper.* – [online] Available from:
http://www.aidsmap.com/en/docs/E7376ADA-92A6-4EA8-852E-BE34FF730A62.asp
[Accessed 18th December 2007].

Wilkie, H. (2007) *Briefing Notes Keep Everyone "In The Loop".* – [online] Available from:
http://ezinearticles.com/?Briefing-Notes-Keep-Everyone-In-The-Loop&id=757512
[Accessed 18th December 2007].

Interprofessional Module 3 – Reflective Essay

The following essay intends to be a reflective piece, which focuses on and examines my own learning and professional development within the context of this module. Throughout this essay the issues raised, which pertain to the subject of interprofessional working will be linked to my current experiences of collaborative education and practice; the ways in which these issues may impact upon my future practice as a qualified healthcare professional will also be discussed. During the course of this module, work was conducted in groups of student healthcare professionals from different disciplines over an online discussion board, following an initial face-to-face meeting; from this work and my subsequent reading, several issues emerged with regard to the needs of professionals in future collaborative practice.

According to Golanowski et al (2007) the improvement of future care delivery "will require" an interprofessional collaborative approach; this widely recognised view is reinforced by their significant assertion that all healthcare professionals possess an "interdependence" upon one another. McGoldrick et al (2001) also argue this viewpoint. This emphasises the need for professionals to collaborate if increasingly complex patient needs are to be successfully addressed, and also reaffirms that very seldom can one professional group achieve the delivery of high quality care alone (Headrick et al, 1998 and Hornby and Atkins, 2000).

However, it is interesting to note that Hammond et al (1999) report that differences in professional education between healthcare professionals of different disciplines means that professionals have "little experience of shared responsibilities" immediately post-registration; adding that this can cause professionals to be reluctant to engage fully with interprofessional practices. One may therefore conclude that interprofessional education, as was experienced and shared within this module across disciplines, will serve to enhance the working interprofessional relationships of those involved (Macleod, 2006). Importantly, the high level of involvement offered to all participants of such interprofessional education is both empowering and "antihierarchical", which may set good foundations for students approaching qualified practice (Lymbery, 2002). Additionally, McGoldrick et al (2001) suggest that

13

interprofessional education is beneficial for students undergoing the "transformation into the leadership role" of a qualified healthcare professional. Once qualified, "high expectations" can be made of healthcare professionals by numerous parties that may be encountered in practice, such as their colleagues and their patients and the relatives of their patients. Furthermore, according to Philpott and Corrigan (2006) being viewed as a role model "cannot be escaped"; and obviously this has clear implications for all student healthcare professionals approaching registration, which should be taken seriously.

The discussions raised within the briefing papers of the interprofessional group highlighted that many students feel overwhelmed and intimidated by the prospect of legally enforced professional accountability, which comes with registration as a qualified professional (Bothamley, 2006). Importantly, Dowling et al (1996) report that the specific roles of healthcare disciplines will "evolve" in order to meet the changing needs of both patients and the healthcare service itself; furthermore Lymbery (2002) adds that professionals are being expected to conduct a "wider range" of duties in their clinical practice. Despite this, Yerbury (1997) reports that although particular duties and responsibilities may change with time, professionals will always remain accountable for their practice. Professionals must be mindful of this, and consequently should be clear about their duties and what is expected of them (Lymbery, 2002; Martin, 2001 and Reid, 2004).

An area of concern relating to professional accountability, particularly for nurses is highlighted by Whitman (2005) suggesting that accountable professionals, whilst having their own responsibilities towards patient care, must also "oversee the duties of others" following the delegating of work to unqualified support staff; adding that when a task has been delegated, the delegating professional is not absolved of accountability for the performance of that task; responsibility for the performance of that task may have been entrusted elsewhere, but not the accountability for the "process or outcome".

Currie and Loftus-Hills (2002) state that the issue of accountability has the potential to conjure up feelings of anxiety and fear within newly qualified professionals, particularly with regard to possible consequences and implications of making difficult decisions. It is for this reason that both Maas (1998) and Macleod (2006) suggest that it is not only good practice for healthcare professionals to thoroughly document their contributions to care in the appropriate patient case notes, but it is essential; this allows professionals to safeguard their professional integrity by providing a record of the justification and rationale for specific care interventions. The dangers of not doing so have been highlighted during my clinical placements where the duplication and omission of work has occurred as a result of patient records being incomplete or inadequate (Yerbury, 1997). Consequently, during future practice I will endeavour to provide detailed and thorough documentation of any care, which I deliver and also the reasons for doing so; I believe that this is a realistic way in which I can employ my learning from the discussions raised within the interprofessional group work for the benefit of future collaborative practice. It may also be worth considering membership of a relevant union for the benefit of legal protection (Dowling et al, 1996).

The initial meeting of the interprofessional group allowed group members to witness the stages of group development first-hand; however, according to Bell (2000) such initial meetings are essential in order for group members to familiarise with the collective goals and purposes of the group. The group in which I was a member, formed quickly following the opening introductions, and all members agreed that thorough planning of the tasks ahead should be take place; significantly, Yerbury (1997) suggests that this was beneficial to the making of progress for the group, as "strategic planning and cooperation are essential" for successful collaboration.

Difficulty was anticipated be some of the participants with regard to communicating via the internet and maintaining an awareness of up-to-date group issues. This is an important issue, as "timely communication" is fundamental to effective collaboration (Macleod, 2006). In addition, Golanowski et al (2007), Hammond et al (1999) and McGoldrick et al (2001) all suggest that the online discussion board may have limited group members in the range of communication skills which could be easily and successfully employed within the group processes and module work. Consequently, it was agreed within the group that all members (wherever possible) were to inspect the online discussion board on a daily basis, in order to ensure that individual members remained up-to-date with regard to the tasks and the progress of others; I feel that this worked well for the group, and such action is advocated by Pringle (2000) who states that interprofessional teams should be "proactive" rather than reactive.

Bell (2000) suggests that the learning-focused climate of the course was conducive to the facilitation and promotion of interprofessional team growth. Following this a "sense of collective responsibility" became apparent at times when others were dependent upon my own personal contribution, in order to make progress (Allen, 2000); I feel that this served to motivate my participation in the collaborative working of the module, particularly when critically appraising the work of my peers; and furthermore, I believe that in my future collaborative practice it will be worthwhile to consider the numerous other parties which may, at times, be relying on my work.

According to Philpott and Corrigan (2006) poor attendance and time keeping is often a significant barrier to successful team working, due to the extra pressure that this can exert on colleagues. The interprofessional group in which I was a member also anticipated this, and subsequently contingency plans were made that in the event of difficulties arising in keeping to the predetermined schedule, then the rest of the group were to be alerted to this as soon as possible. One of the emerging themes from the work produced by the group, was that "tensions" and "conflicts" between different accountabilities can arise (Allen, 2000); however it may be interesting to note that such a conflict of duties was experienced during the course of this module, as I was not only accountable for the completion of the work for this module, but was also accountable for the completion of work elsewhere.

The group work also highlighted a need for teams to be "open to change" (Bell, 2000). This became evident when instructions for the critical appraisal of the work of other group members were changed at an intermediate stage of the module; this caused some confusion initially, but did not provide any lasting problems. Similarly, in practice interprofessional teams must be prepared for unexpected changes, for example at times when the condition or status of a patient and their condition may change. The initial contingency planning and agreed rules for the group allowed itself to function when these changes occurred, as all members kept in regular contact, and actively participated and shared information; this proved to be beneficial and I will aim to adopt such stringent and consistent approaches when working collaboratively in future practice.

All group members were required to actively participate in the devising of a framework with which to guide the critiquing of briefing papers produced by other group members (included as an appendix). McGoldrick et al (2001) report that "participation in decision making" is beneficial for team member morale; this view is reinforced by Bell (2000) who reports that the involving of team members in decision making processes is empowering, and can lead to improved results and a "sense of accomplishment" when completing tasks. These findings were echoed within my interprofessional group, with a number of students describing feelings of empowerment with regard to devising a tool, which would guide their future work.

The "supportive environment" and respect fostered within the interprofessional module group enabled critical feedback from other group members to be given, and promotes "critical reflection" in clinical practice (McGoldrick et al, 2001). Being the recipient of such feedback provided a good opportunity to gather constructive advice from my peers regarding my contributions to the interprofessional collaborative group efforts; this allowed me to modify my approach and technique when tackling the subsequent tasks. In future practice I predict that it will be beneficial for me to consider such constructive feedback from colleagues in order to improve my performance. Furthermore, Bell (2000) states that "feedback from team members" fosters interprofessional growth, whilst McGoldrick et al (2001) add that such "recognition by colleagues" improves morale and performance.

Clouder and Sellars (2004) argue that "interprofessional supervision" allows the "full potential" of reflective practice to be recognised "more readily"; therefore, one may assume that the benefits of participating in this module may be multifaceted. Additionally, McGoldrick et al (2001) state that reflection can have a "significant impact" on the subsequent experiences of an individual, which suggests that the work of this module could potentially have a widespread positive impact on my future practice and also that of the other participants (Cloud and Sellars, 2004). Furthermore, McGoldrick et al (2001) add that "team learning" is beneficial for interprofessional practice as it "encourages collaboration".

There is much literature advocating the use of interprofessional approaches to practice (Headrick et al, 1998 and Holmes, 2003). However, according to Hammond et al (1999) views of "unilateral" working continue to be favoured by a minority of professionals, which can present difficulties in collaborative practice; although this was not overtly evident during the group work of this module. I predict that in the future of the modern healthcare service, the NHS will be increasingly required to work with and alongside the private healthcare sector; this notion is supported by Currie and Loftus-Hills (2002), and as a result they assert that there will be an increased need to develop improved interprofessional "partnerships" in years to come. The role of interprofessional collaboration in the modern healthcare system is both key and unquestionable; however I feel that by participating in this module I have been provided with a direct opportunity to experience some of the processes involved personally. This will be beneficial to my future practice, and will allow my collaborative working approach to "mature" from a "multidisciplinary" one, to an "interdisciplinary" one (Yerbury, 1997).

Word count – 2008.

Reference List

Allen, P. (2000) Accountability for clinical governance: developing collective responsibility for quality in primary care. *British Medical Journal* 321(7261) p.608-611.

Bell, H. (2000) Shared governance and teamwork-myth or reality. *AORN* 71(3) p.631, 632, 634, 635.

Bothamley, J. (2006) Face up to responsibility. *Nursing Standard* 20(45) p.77.

Clouder, L. and Sellars, J. (2004) Reflective practice and clinical supervision: an interprofessional perspective. *Journal of Advanced Nursing* 46(3) p.262–269.

Currie, L. and Loftus-Hills, A. (2002) The nursing view of clinical governance. *Nursing Standard* 16(27) p.40-44.

Dowling, S., Martin, R., Skidmore, P., Doyal, L., Cameron, A. and Lloyd, S. (1996) Nurses taking on junior doctors' work: a confusion of accountability. *British Medical Journal* 312(7040) p.1211-1214.

Golanowski, M., Beaudry, D., Kurz, L., Laffey, W. and Hook, M. (2007) Interdisciplinary Shared Decision-Making: Taking Shared Governance to the Next Level. *Nursing Administration Quarterly* 31(4) p.341–353.

Hammond, K., Bandak, A. and Williams, M. (1999) Nurse, Physician, and Consumer Role Responsibility Perceived by Health Care Providers. *Holistic Nursing Practice* 13(2) p.28-37.

Headrick, L., Wilcock, P. and Batalden, P. (1998) Continuing medical education: Interprofessional working and continuing medical education. *British Medical Journal* 316(7133) p.771-774.

Holmes, S. (2003) Undernutrition in hospital patients. *Nursing Standard* 17(19) p.45-52, 54-55.

Hornby, S. and Atkins, J. (2000) *Collaborative Care: Interprofessional, Interagency and Interpersonal.* 2nd ed, Oxford: Blackwell Science.

Lymbery, M. (2002) Shared governance in the community. *Journal of Nursing Management* 10(5) p.291–298.

Maas, M. (1998) Nursing's Role in Interdisciplinary Accountability for Patient Outcomes. *Outcomes Management for Nursing Practice* 2(3) p.92-94.

Macleod, A. (2006) The nursing role in preventing delay in patient discharge. *Nursing Standard* 21(1) p.43-48.

Martin, V. (2001) Service planning and governance: Part Two: Managing accountability and risk. *Nursing Management* 8(3) p.33-37.

McGoldrick, T., Menschner, E. and Pollock, M. (2001) Nurturing the Transformation from Staff Nurse to Leader. *Holistic Nursing Practice* 16(1) p.16–20.

Philpott, S. and Corrigan, P. (2006) Role modelling. *Nursing Management* 13(1) p.10-12.

Pringle, M. (2000) Participating in clinical governance. *British Medical Journal* 321(7263) p.737-740.

Reid, W. (2004) Organization Liability: Beyond *Respondeat Superior. Journal of Psychiatric Practice* 10(4) p.258-262.

Whitman, M. (2005) Return and Report: Establishing accountability in delegation. *American Journal of Nursing* 105(3) p.97.

Yerbury, M. (1997) Issues in multidisciplinary teamwork for children with disabilities. *Child: Care, Health and Development* 23(1) p.77–86.

Critique Criteria

1. What is the main focus of the briefing paper?
   - Is there a sentence that states the main purpose or focus of the paper?
   - How well does the paper focus on the main topic?

2. Is the aim of the paper clear and concise (easy to understand, not excessively verbose)?
   - Is it clear what the writer is trying to accomplish?
   - Does the paper inform, persuade, explain or entertain?
   - Is the purpose of the paper appropriate for the audience?
   - Are the important terms clearly defined?

3. Is the intended audience of the briefing paper clear?
   - Does it take into account the readers previous experience and knowledge?
   - Does it contain information that will interest the reader?
   - Are the vocabulary, tone and style of the paper appropriate for the chosen audience?

4. What evidence does the writer use to support their point of view?
   - Does the writer provide sufficient convincing evidence to support their arguments?
   - Does the author provide a balanced view? If a biased view is presented does the author provide a reasonable argument?
   - Are any assumptions made?
   - Has the author used evidence from a range of different sources?

5. Does the writer use sufficient appropriate references to support their work?

6. Is the referencing of supporting material clear and in keeping with the 'Harvard Referencing' system?
   - Is there a reference list?
   - Does this match the references in the briefing paper?

7. Has the paper explored at least one of the module themes (governance, user participation or collaborative working)?
   - What themes have emerged, and are they appropriate?

8. Does the writer challenge any arguments and ideas, or suggest ways in which things may be improved?
   - What issues are raised?
   - Are the arguments justified?
   - Are there any opposing views presented?
   - Does the writer provide evidence of ethical consideration in the paper?

9. Is there a clear summary, and does the writer demonstrate that they have learned something from the discussion?
   - What was your overall impression of the paper?
   - Were discussions presented in an interesting form?
   - Does the author fulfil the stated purpose of the paper?
   - Has your knowledge been enhanced by reading the paper?
   - Do you agree with the findings?

10. Does the paper meet the learning outcomes?
    - Have the factors that impact on the quality of health and social care provision been discussed?

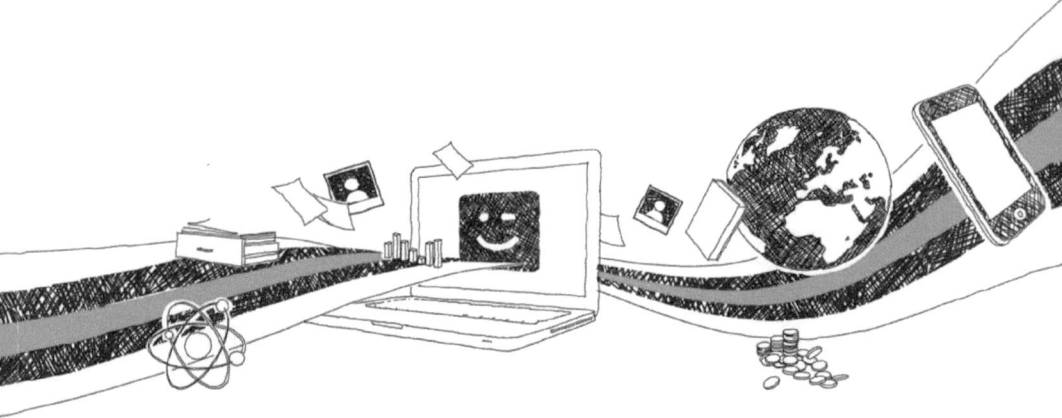
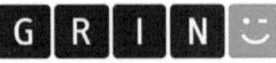